Last Goodbye

Poems for Transitions

Last Goodbye

Poems for Transitions

David Lee Woods

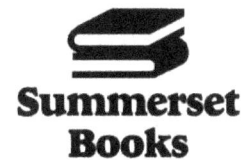

Summerset Books

Last Goodbye
Poems for Transitions

David Lee Woods

Editors:
Veronica Mabel Woods
Scott Walter Woods
Mia Catherine Chambers
Phyllis Dorathy Chambers
Ruth Schwartz

© 2015 by David Lee Woods. All rights reserved.

ISBN: 978-09715509-4-0 (Paperback Large Print)
ISBN: 978-09715509-5-7 (eBook)

Cover photograph by the author.
Illustrations licensed from:
 Can Stock Photos Inc. and Shutterstock Inc.
Published by: Summerset Books, Walnut Creek CA
Printed in the United States of America.

Dedicated to Mary Jane and Phyllis, our extended families, and all those who are struggling with transitions after a loss.

To help keep family memories alive there is a blank page after each poem so that the reader can make notes about related experiences.

Contents

Getting Old ix
Wondering 1
    The Vigil 2
    Emergency Room 4
    Consultation Room 6
    The Long Hall 8
    The Cry 10
    A Beautiful Sound 14
    The Phone Call 16
    Holding Tight 18
    Words Remembered 20
    The Gurney 22
Passing 25
    The Blocked Path 26
    Finally 28
    Watching Him Work 30
    My Brother 32

When the Bells Rang	34
Past Tense	36
Home at Last	38
A Quick Hello	40
Remembering	**43**
The Usual	44
Our Song	46
Alone Again	48
Oh Do I Miss You	50
A Year Ago	52
Alone	56
Safe Anchorage	58
Last Goodbye	61
About the Book	**65**
About the Author	**66**
Books by Author	**67**
List of Poems	**68**

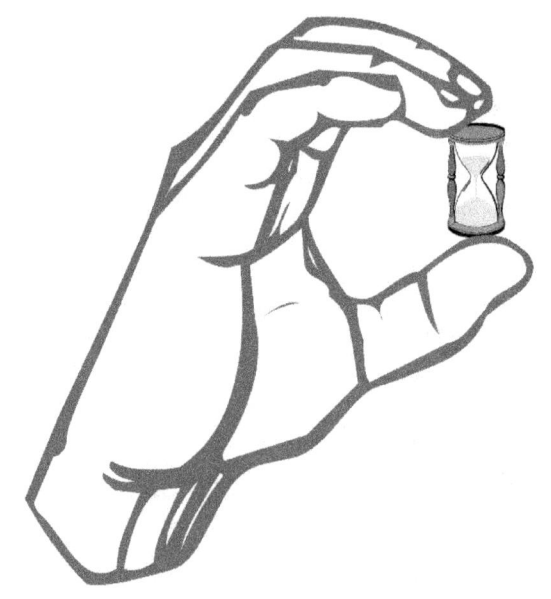

Getting Old

I stopped wondering
    if I looked old
when a young woman
    got up to give me
        her seat.

Memories about starting to feel old.

x

Memories about starting to feel old.

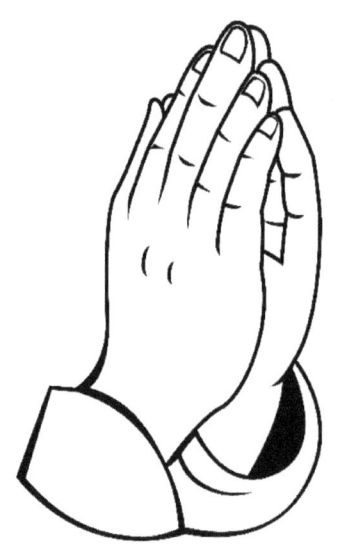

Wondering

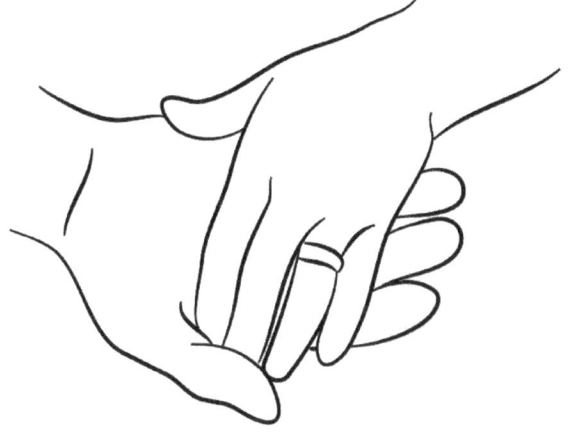

The Vigil

In the darkened church
    we held hands
as we watched families
    carrying lit candles
to put by photographs of
    departed loved ones.

We were each wondering
    when one of us
would take our turn in that line
    of families going forward
to place our lit candle
    by the other's photograph.

Memories of wondering about death.

Emergency Room

Though we are
    here together,
We are alone
    within ourselves,
Wondering what
    might be.

Memories of medical emergencies.

Consultation Room

The rooms were all full
    and gurneys lined the hall.

Her gurney was by a sign that
    read Consultation Room.

I was glad to be standing there
    waiting and not sitting

In that room — with a doctor,
    and the door closed.

Memories of waiting for a doctor.

The Long Hall

She walked down the long hall.
    And Oh! So very long it was.

She walked with quickened pace
    staring straight ahead.

Her face somber
    as tears welled up.

I dared not look —
    I did not want to see her cry.

Memories of watching others in anguish.

The Cry

As we waited, I watched more
    gurneys go past her room.

I half dozed as I sat there,
    watching her rest.

I was lulled by the sound of
    muted medical talk,

Punctuated by the
    "bings" and "bongs"
    of medical equipment.

Then — I was jolted wide awake
    by the sound every
    parent knows:

That unforgettable sound of a
    baby's piercing cry.

And I was flooded with the
    memories of our children

So many years ago —
    when they were small

And I carried them into
    the Emergency Room.

Memories of children and hospitals.

Memories of children and hospitals.

A Beautiful Sound

I sat there by her bed
watching her sleep,
oh so quiet and still.

I listened to her breathing,
oh such a beautiful sound.

Memories of wandering
what will happen next.

The Phone Call

Doctor?

Test results!

Come now?

Bring wife?

Memories about the unknown.

Holding Tight

As I sat there
she gripped my hand
as if she was trying
to hold on to life itself.

Memories about sharing anxiety.

Words Remembered

We told the doctor
    that we were all there.

He told us
    what we did not want to hear.

Medical terms
    were hard to understand.

But just a few
    I will not soon forget.

Like terminal cancer
    and hospice care.

Memories about the dreaded truth.

The Gurney

She lay there
    on the gurney
As we waited
    for the doctor.
As I watched
    her breathe
Each breath so
    very slow
I dared not
    look away
For fear her breath
    would stop
And I would
    not act
        in time.

Memories of anxious waiting.

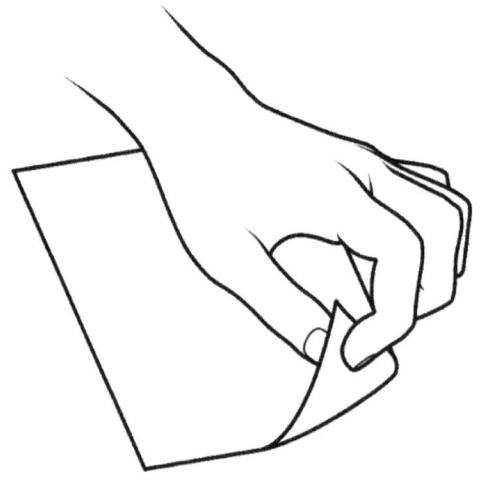

Passing

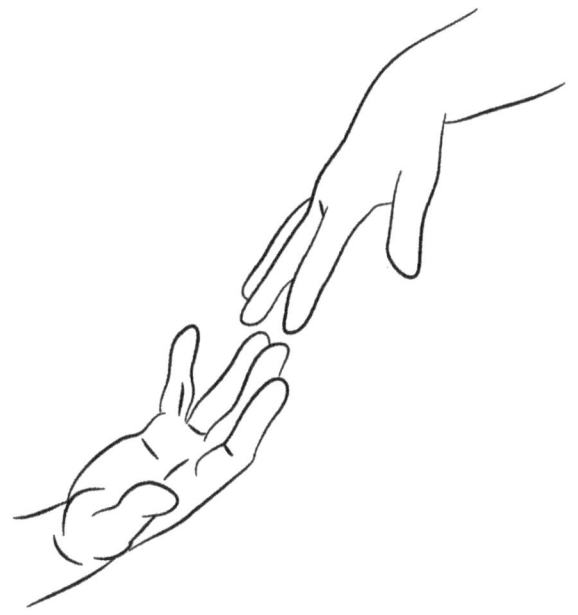

The Blocked Path

There is a path to where
    we do not know,

A path that we must
    each walk alone.

When the gate opens
    on that blocked path,

We become but
    cherished memories
        for those we leave behind.

Memories about wondering who will remember.

Finally

As he had requested,
he was at home
under hospice care.

He was comfortable
and not in pain.

He talked all evening
with his family
as his cat purred in his lap.

As he listened to his
favorite Beatles music,
he closed his eyes
and stopped breathing.

Memories about dying.

Watching Him Work

He covers a mound of dirt
    with a green drape.
Puts twelve chairs
    in two neat rows,
Lays a green drape
    by the open grave.

Soon all will be ready for
    the hearse and the family.
As I watch him work
    I wonder how long it will be,
until he will need
    to get everything ready
        — for me.

Memories about cemetery visits.

My Brother

There was a hurt so long ago,
    a hurt I never did forgive.
I gave him not my love again
    and let a chill come
        in between.
But here with these strangers
    I see his casket
        resting there.
I hear so many tell of a friend,
    a man so full
        of loving care.
I hear them all tell
    about a man, a brother
        I wish I had known.

Memories about family relations.

When the Bells Rang

The sun glistened
    from dew drops
        on fresh-cut grass.
And mourning doves
    hopped around the stone
        looking for food.
The jays chattered
    high in the trees
        at my approach.
In the soft hush
    the calling of
        the birds was clear.
Like the church bells
    the day
        I laid my love to rest.

Memories about funerals.

Past Tense

When I heard *"I baptize thee,"*
    I thought of a future with oh
    so much to look forward to.

When I heard *"I now thee wed,"*
    I thought about our past
    then of their future together.

When I heard *"Now rest in peace,"*
    I could only think of the past
    for now there is no future.

Memories about a family death.

Home at Last

The fresh-dug sod
    has settled now,
And the
    headstone's sheen
        has faded.
Grass
    now covers
        the stone's sharp edge,
As the earth
    makes the stone
        a home —
Like my love
    at rest there now
        in the good earth
            from which she came.

Memories of cemetery visits.

A Quick Hello

I came by to say
    a quick hello.
But I will not stay
    for long.
For I have things
    I need to do.

But I know that I
    will be back.
And some day it will
    be to stay.
Here in the plot
    next to yours.

Memories of cemetery visits.

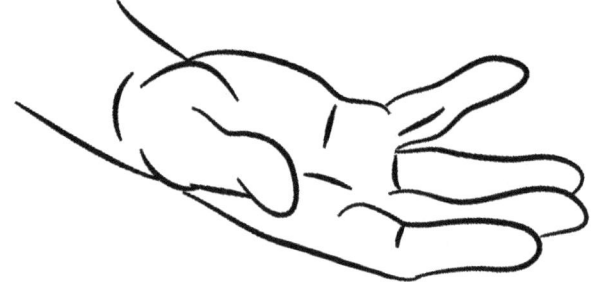

42

Remembering

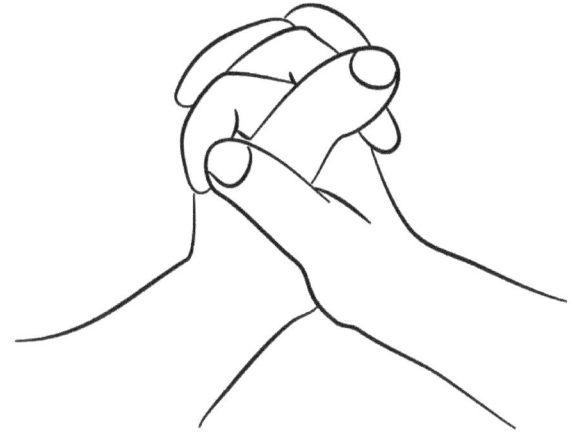

The Usual

The usual greeting
    but — different.

Hospital bed,
    medical stuff —
        gone.

From now on
    there will be
        a new usual.

Memories about visiting.

Our Song

I heard our song
    and I said —
        remember when?

But silence answered,
    she was not there —
        she had slipped away.

Memories about remembering when.

Alone Again

She wasn't there
    to say goodbye
        as she always had.
I turned off the lights
    and locked the door
        then went on my way.
She had turned our house
    into a home, but now
        it is just a house again.
Our things are all
    still here, but
        the love is gone.
The house is now
    like my heart,
        dark and cold.
I feel so empty
    with nothing left
        but memories.

Memories about feeling alone.

Oh Do I Miss You

Oh do I miss you
    in the morning
    when the coffee is
    brewing strong.

Oh do I miss you
    in the evening
    when the day
    has been so long.

Oh to hear you say
    "It'll be okay."
    Oh yes, I miss you
    every single day.

Memories about feeling alone.

A Year Ago

Last year I knew
     the joys of deep love,
     as we dreamed together
     of our tomorrows.

Then, just a year ago
     my world fell apart;
     now I stand alone
     looking at your stone.

Since my last visit
     to this quiet place,
     you have a new neighbor
     under fresh-dug sod.

There are those of us
     who come here to visit,
     to show our respect
     and just remember.

But for us, our lives
    must go on each day;
    we too must have
    new neighbors near us.

We now share our lives
    with others we know.
    Lives are for the living;
    cemeteries for the dead.

I will never forget you,
    but I must go on.
    Goodbye, my love,
    and rest in peace.

Memories about starting to move on.

Memories about starting to move on.

Alone

Candle's flame
    and soft music,
a place set for one —
    a glass filled for
        a long night ahead.

Memories about
accepting being alone.

Safe Anchorage

May your anchorage
    always be sheltered
    from the storm.

And in the early morning mist
    may you hear the fish jump
    and the birds sing softly.

And may the sun fill
    your heart
    as it does the day
    with warmth.

Memories about starting to move on.

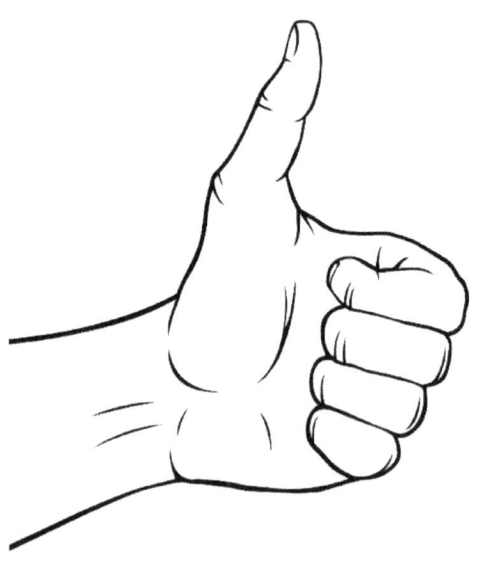

Last Goodbye

When they come by
to say their last goodbye
they will see me in
my favorite suit and tie.
Sure hope they'll say,
"Looks good for an old guy."

Memories of wondering about death.

Memories of thinking about what is next.

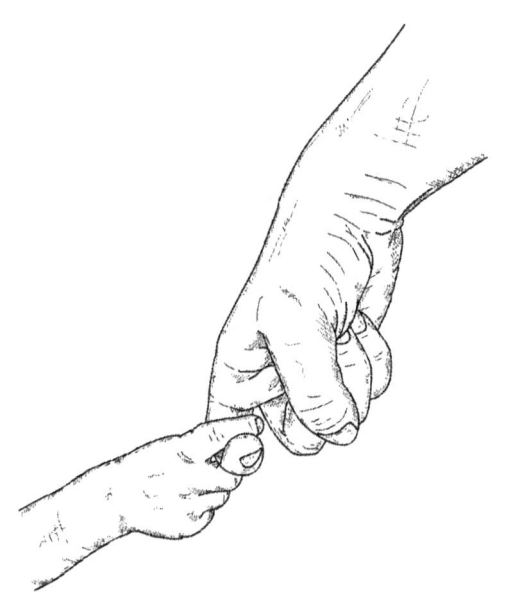

About the Book

This is a collection of poems about what the author saw in the mirrors of his soul as he went through the transitions of living with his extended family and of losing his wife, other family members and friends.

The author hopes that those who are struggling with transitions after a loss will find comfort in these poems and that they will help in sharing experiences.

To help keep family memories alive there is a blank page after each poem so that the reader can make notes about related experiences.

About the Author

The author has been a laborer, manager, researcher, a primary and secondary teacher, and a professor in human resources and occupational health and safety.

    The coupling of his work experience and living with a large extended family has helped him develop an interest in writing nonfiction about management and history, along with writing essays, short stories and poetry.

    These poems come from his experience of losing his wife, other family members and friends. Poetry has been his way of making sense of the world. He hopes that these poems find a response with the reader.

Books by Author

Woods, David Lee (2007). *Change Without Chaos: A Practical Guide to Decision Management.* Philadelphia, PA: Xlibris, Random House

Woods, David Lee (2003). *Cruising Historic San Francisco Bay with FDR's Presidential Yacht Potomac.* Walnut Creek, CA: Summerset Books.

Woods, David Lee (1985). *The Wanderings of My Naked Soul.* Oakland, CA: Private printing.

Woods, David Lee (1980). *My Job, My Boss, and Me.* Belmont, CA: Lifetime Learning, A division of Wadsworth.

List of Poems

A Beautiful Sound 14
A Quick Hello 40
A Year Ago 52
Alone 56
Alone Again 48
Consultation Room 6
Emergency Room 4
Finally 28
Getting Old ix
Holding Tight 18
Home at Last 38
Last Goodbye 61
My Brother 32
Oh Do I Miss You 50

Our Song..*46*
Past Tense *36*
Safe Anchorage *58*
The Blocked Path...............................*26*
The Cry *10*
The Gurney...*22*
The Long Hall..*8*
The Phone Call....................................*16*
The Usual *44*
The Vigil..*2*
Watching Him Work..........................*30*
When the Bells Rang *34*
Words Remembered *20*

www.ingramcontent.com/pod-product-compliance
Lightning Source LLC
Chambersburg PA
CBHW070629050426
42450CB00011B/3145